Dear Ones,

If you're going through a difficult time in your life, know that you're not alone. Everyone faces challenges at some point, and it's important to remember that these struggles can make us stronger and more resilient.

One way to cope with difficult emotions and find peace during the dark night of the soul is through coloring. Coloring has been shown to have a calming effect on the mind and can help reduce stress and anxiety.

When you color, you can focus on the task and let go of any negative thoughts or worries weighing you down. The simple act of filling in the lines and choosing colors can be a meditative experience, allowing you to let go of your troubles and find some inner peace.

So if you're feeling overwhelmed or lost during the dark night of the soul, consider taking some time to color. It may seem small, but it can make a big difference in how you feel and cope with your struggles. Allow yourself to take a break and focus on something simple and enjoyable. You may be surprised at the benefits it can bring to your mental health and well-being.

Trust the process

Trust the process, though it's hard to see,
The winding path that lies ahead of thee,
For in the midst of darkness and despair,
There is a light, a hope that's always there.

The road may twist, and turn, and wind,
But trust the journey that you're on, my friend,
For every step, though it may be tough,
Will lead you to a place that's good enough.

Though the path may be steep and rough,
And doubts may linger and call your bluff,
Believe in yourself, and you will find,
The strength to keep going, and leave doubts behind.

Trust the process, though it may be slow,
The destination is worth the journey, though.
For in the end, you'll find your way,
And shine as bright as the light of day.

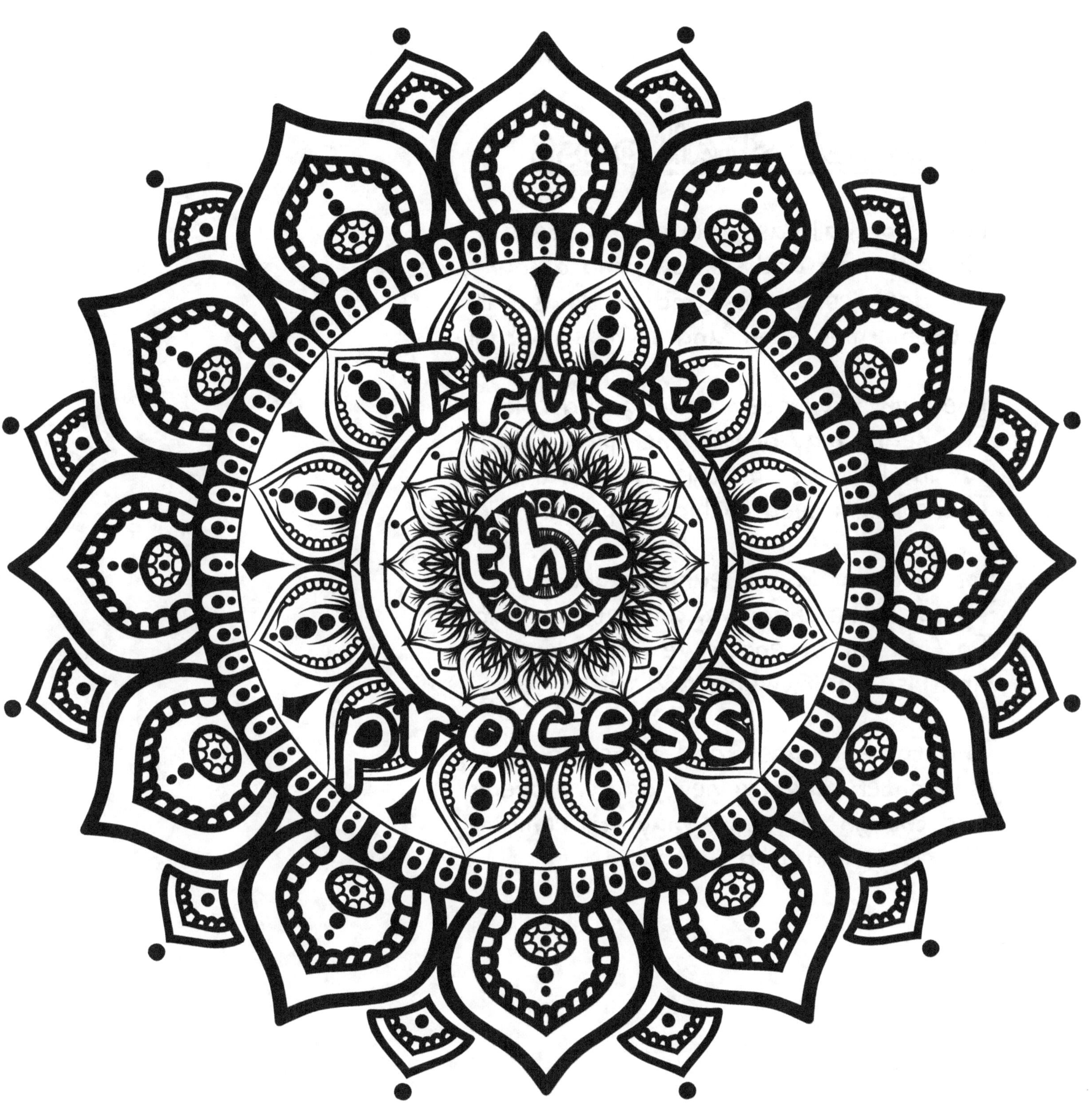

Trust
the
process

This too shall pass

This too shall pass, the saying goes,
Through pain and sorrow, and all our woes,
The darkness comes, and shadows fall,
But time moves on, and so must we all.

The night may seem so long and cold,
The heart may break, the spirit fold,
But in the midst of this dark hour,
There lies a seed of hidden power.

For in the pain, we learn to grow,
To face the shadows, and let them go,
To find the strength we never knew,
And rise again, whole and anew.

This too shall pass, and in its wake,
A brighter dawn, a new day will break,
And though the scars may still remain,
We rise again, and live again.

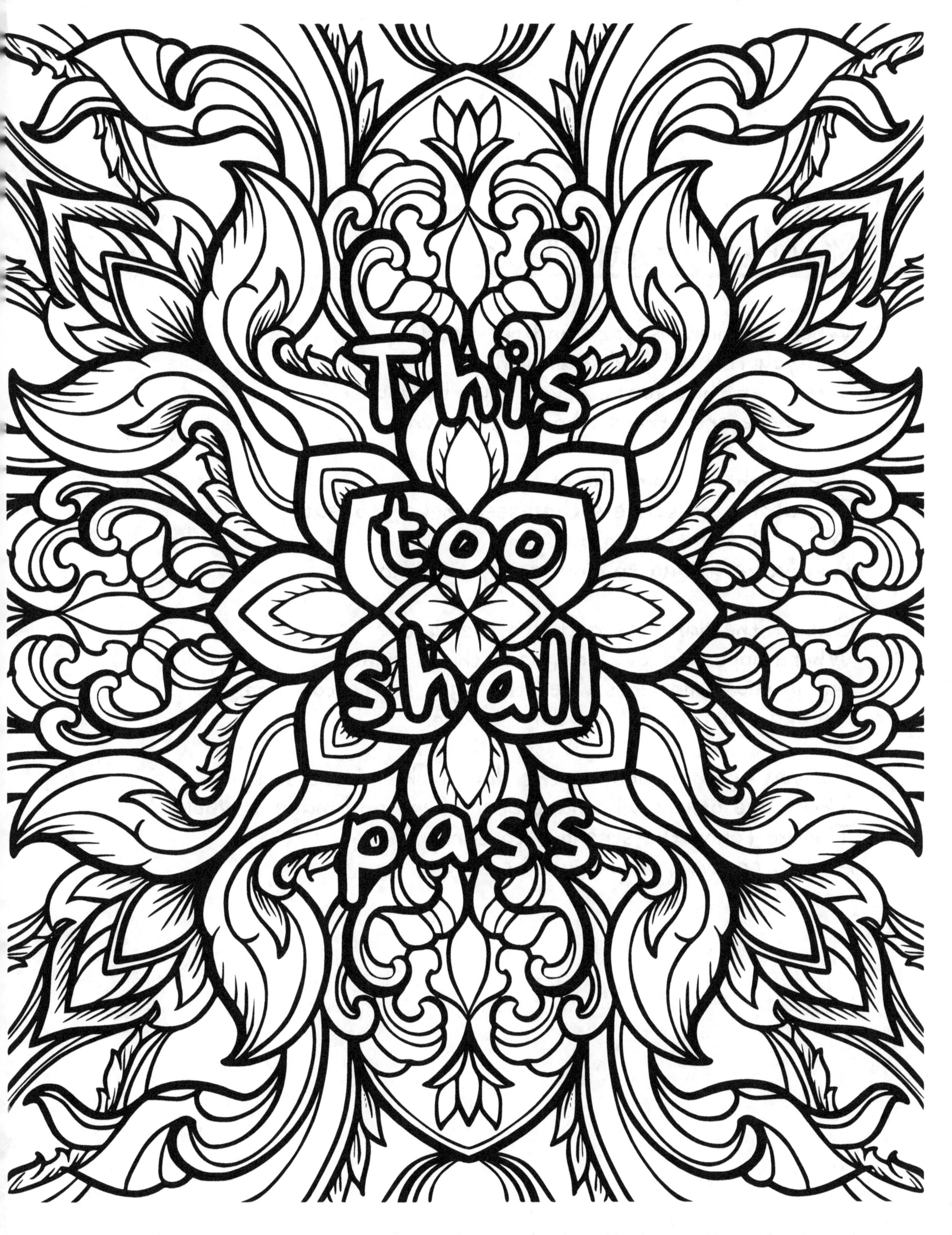
This
too
shall
pass

You are not alone

When the night is dark and the road is long,
And you feel like you're all alone,
Remember that you're never truly by yourself,
For there are others who have known.

The weight of pain, the sting of grief,
The depths of sadness that seem never to leave,
We've all felt them in our time,
And we've all had to find a way to climb.

Out of the darkness and into the light,
Where hope and love can make things right,
But in those moments when the night seems too long,
It's okay to feel like you don't belong.

For you are not alone in this dark night of the soul,
There are others who have been there and made it whole,
They've found the strength to carry on,
And so can you, you're just as strong.

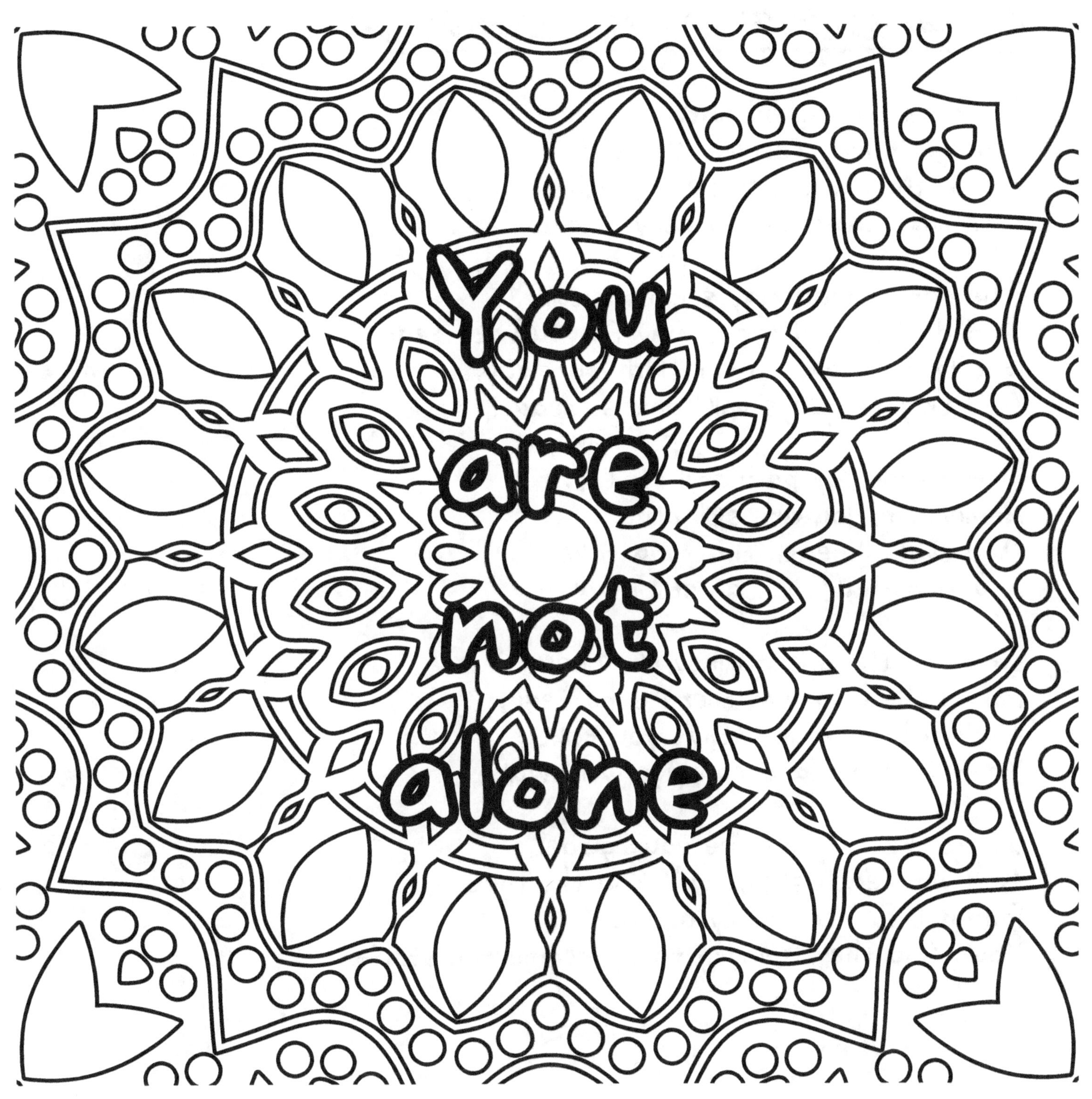

You
are
not
alone

<u>Embrace the uncertainty</u>

Embrace the uncertainty, my friend,
Though it may feel like the end,
For in the darkness there is light,
And hope can shine so very bright.

The path ahead may seem unclear,
And doubts and fears may fill you with fear,
But trust that you will find your way,
And brighter days will come someday.

In the midst of pain and strife,
Remember, you are still alive,
And every breath that you take,
Is a sign that you can still awake.

Embrace the uncertainty, my dear,
For in the unknown there is no fear,
And with each step that you take,
Your strength and courage will awake.

So let the darkness be your guide,
And with each step, you'll find the light,
For in the uncertainty of life,
You'll find the strength to overcome the strife.

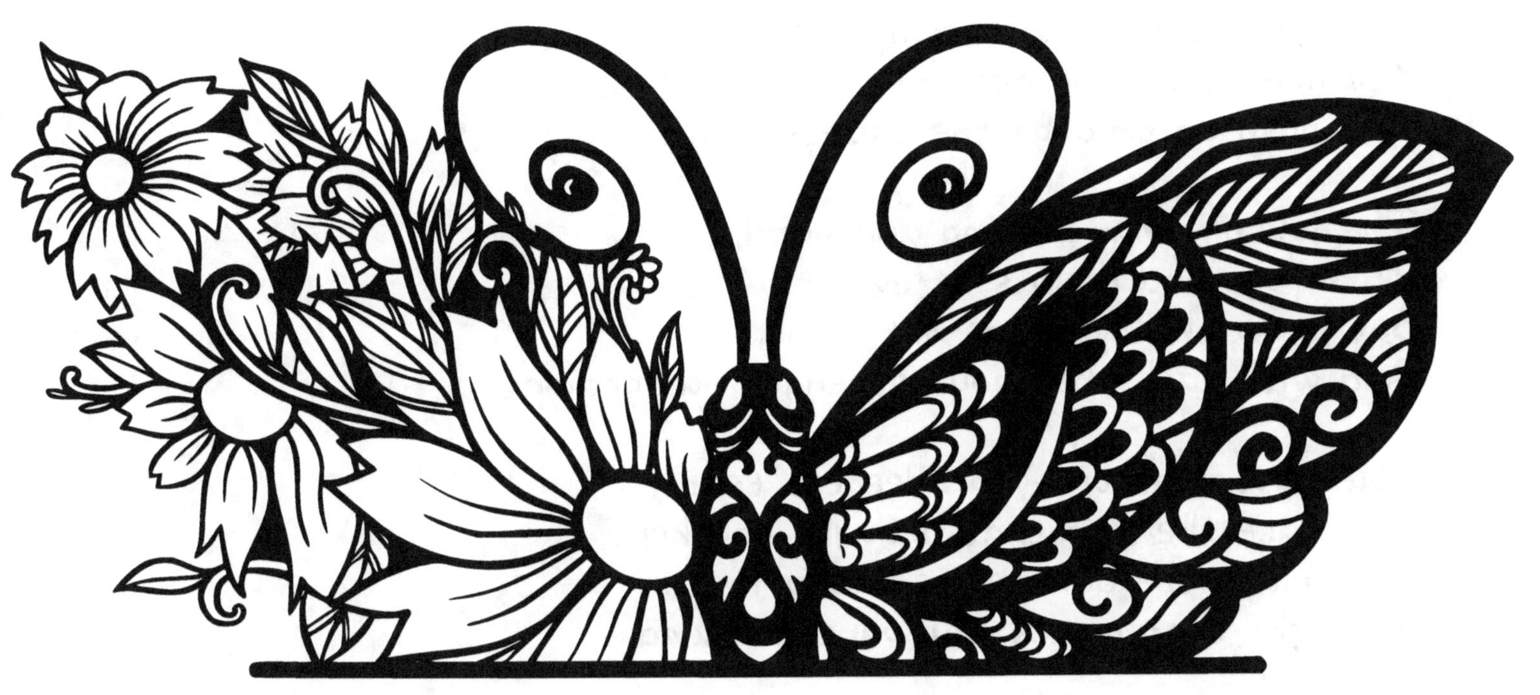

Embrace the uncertainty

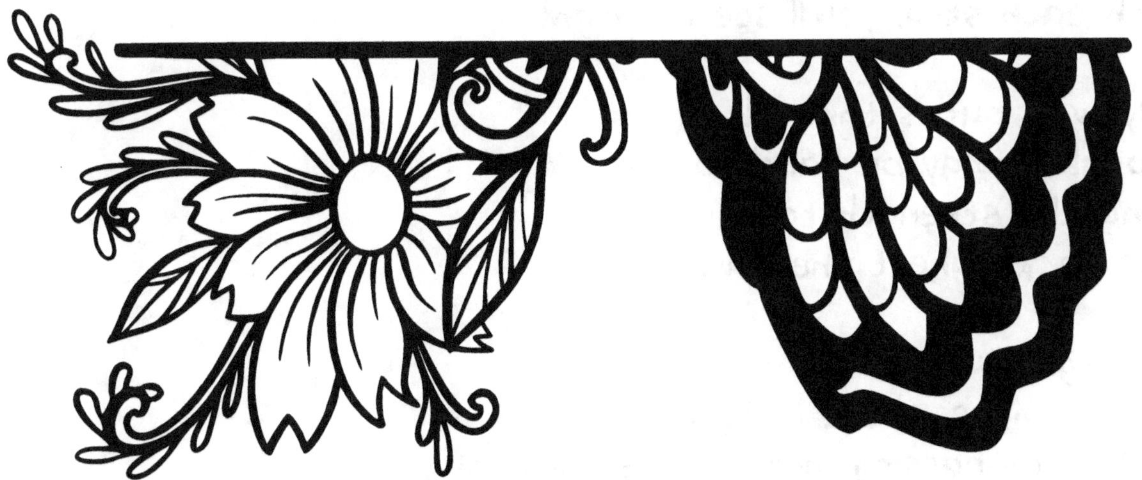

The only way is through

The only way out is through,
Though the path may seem askew,
You must face the dark with light,
And push on through the endless night.

The journey may be long and hard,
With pain and doubts at every yard,
But know that you are not alone,
And with each step, your strength has grown.

You must confront your deepest fears,
And face the pain that brought you here,
For only in the darkness can you find,
The light that guides you, pure and kind.

So keep on moving, step by step,
And do not falter, do not wept,
For in the darkness there is light,
And with each step, you'll see it bright.

The only way out is through,
And though it may be hard to do,
You'll find the strength to carry on,
And rise up, to greet the dawn.

So do not give up, do not despair,
For there is hope, there is repair,
And with each passing moment, please know,
That healing waits, and love will grow.

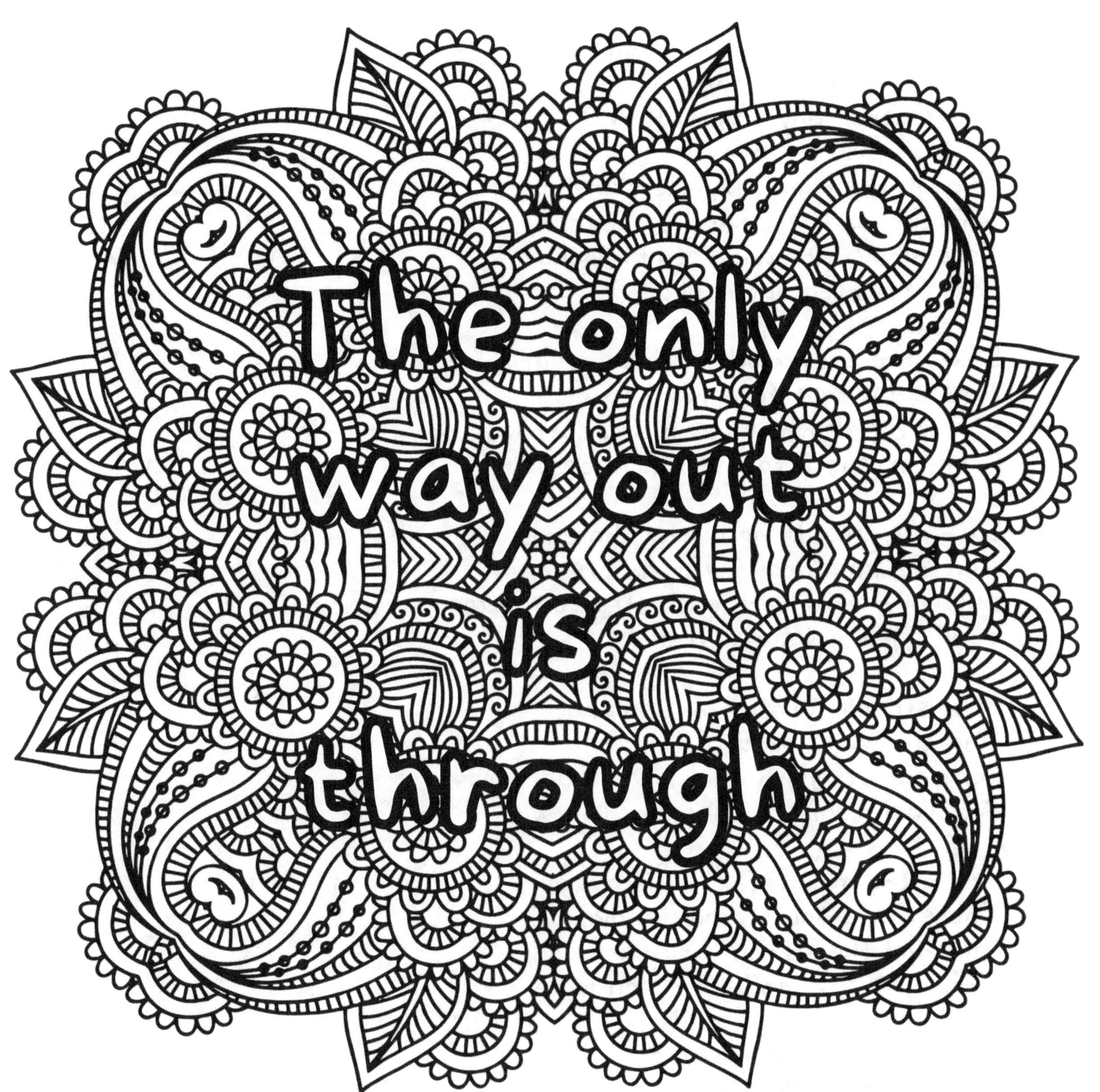

The only
way out
is
through

<u>Stay strong even when it's tough</u>

Stay strong even when it's tough,
And the path ahead is rough,
For within you lies the power,
To weather any stormy hour.

Though the night may seem unending,
And the darkness hard to bear,
Keep your faith and keep believing,
For a brighter day is near.

Stay strong even when you're weary,
And the weight feels hard to bear,
For in the depths of pain and sorrow,
Is the strength to rise above despair.

Each day may bring a new challenge,
And the road may twist and turn,
But know that with each step you take,
Your spirit will surely burn.

Stay strong even when it's hard,
And the way ahead is dim,
For your strength will light the darkness,
And your courage will carry you within.

For in the midst of every struggle,
There's a chance to rise above,
And find the strength to carry on,
Through faith, and hope, and love.

So stay strong, my dear one,
And let your spirit shine,
For in the midst of every storm,
You'll find the light divine.

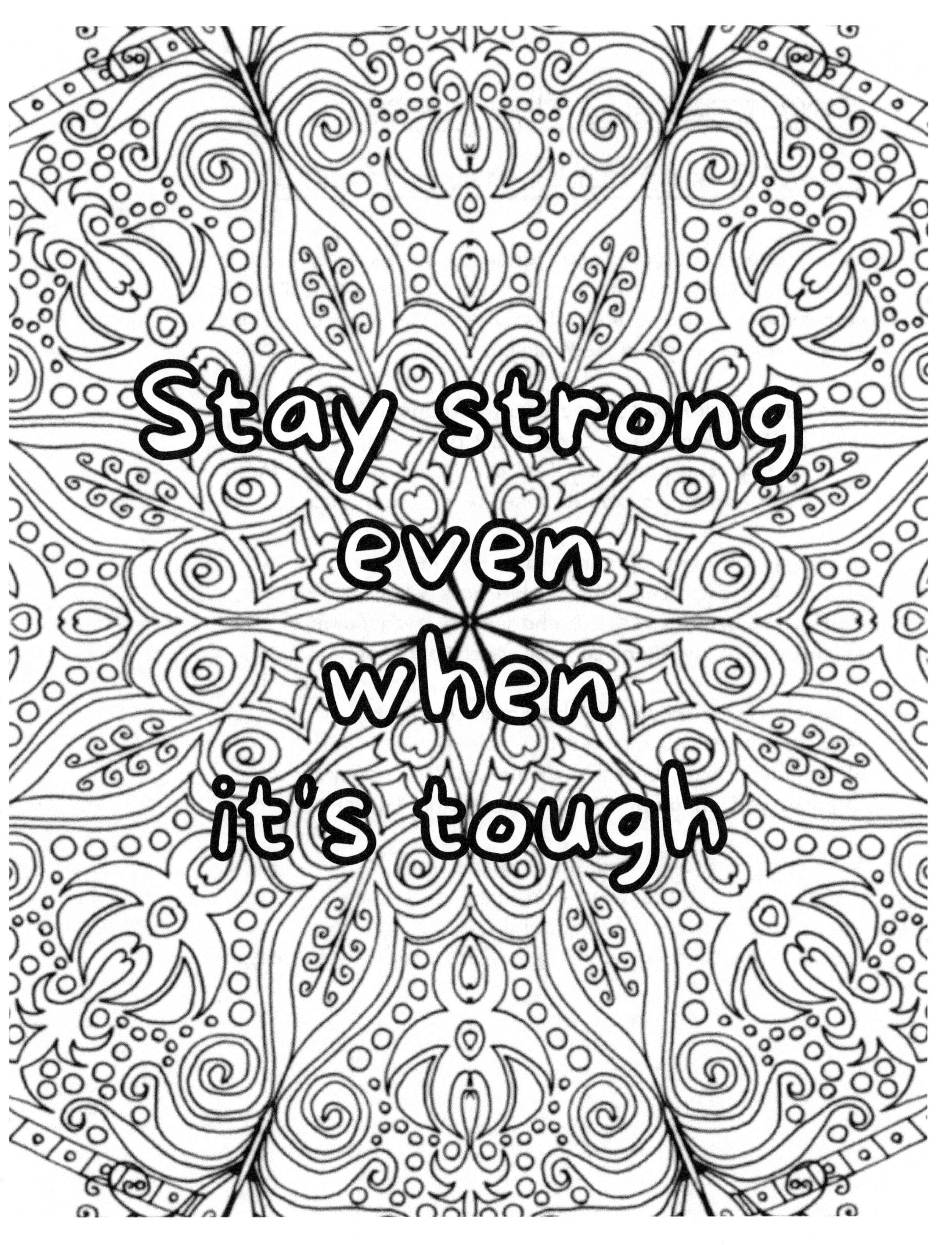

Stay strong
even
when
it's tough

The wound is the place where the light enters you

In the depths of your soul, when all seems lost,
And the weight of the world feels like an impossible cost,
Remember that the wound is where the light can shine,
A glimmer of hope, a new design.

Though the darkness may seem all-consuming,
The light within you is constantly blooming,
And though the pain may feel like it will never cease,
The light can bring about a sense of inner peace.

So let go of control, surrender to the flow,
And trust that the light within you will always grow,
For in the wound lies the chance to transform,
A chance to awaken, to heal, and to reform.

Though the journey may be tough and long,
And at times you may feel completely wronged,
Remember that the light within you will never fade,
Guiding you through the darkness and the shade.

So embrace the wound, let it guide you,
To the path that's true and right and anew,
For in the midst of every trial,
Lies a chance to let your light shine bright and smile.

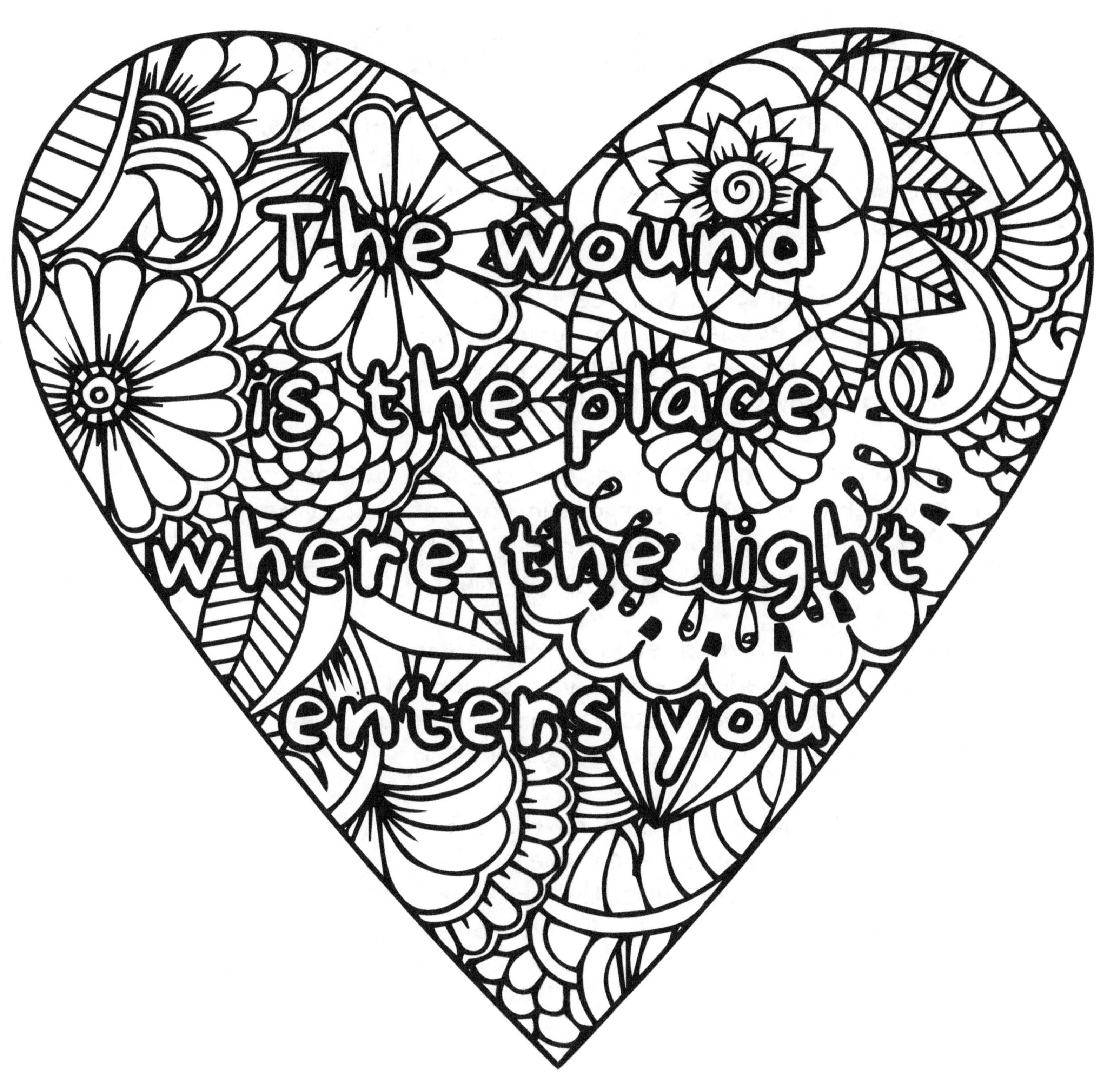

The wound
is the place
where the light
enters you

The deeper the darkness the brighter the light shines

The deeper the darkness, the brighter the light shines,
For even in the blackest of nights, hope still aligns,
A flicker of light that guides you through,
And leads you to a strength you never knew.

In the midst of despair, you feel so alone,
As if the world has left you on your own,
But deep within you, a fire still burns,
A light that grows with every lesson learned.

The darkness can be daunting, and the road unclear,
But know that there's a purpose in each and every tear,
For even in the midst of the darkest night,
The light still shines with a powerful might.

So keep moving forward, even when it's tough,
And know that the light within you is more than enough,
For the deeper the darkness, the brighter you'll shine,
And through it all, you'll rise and you'll climb.

So let the light guide you through the storm,
And trust in the journey, even when it feels forlorn,
For the deeper the darkness, the brighter the light,
And in that light, you'll find your way out of the night.

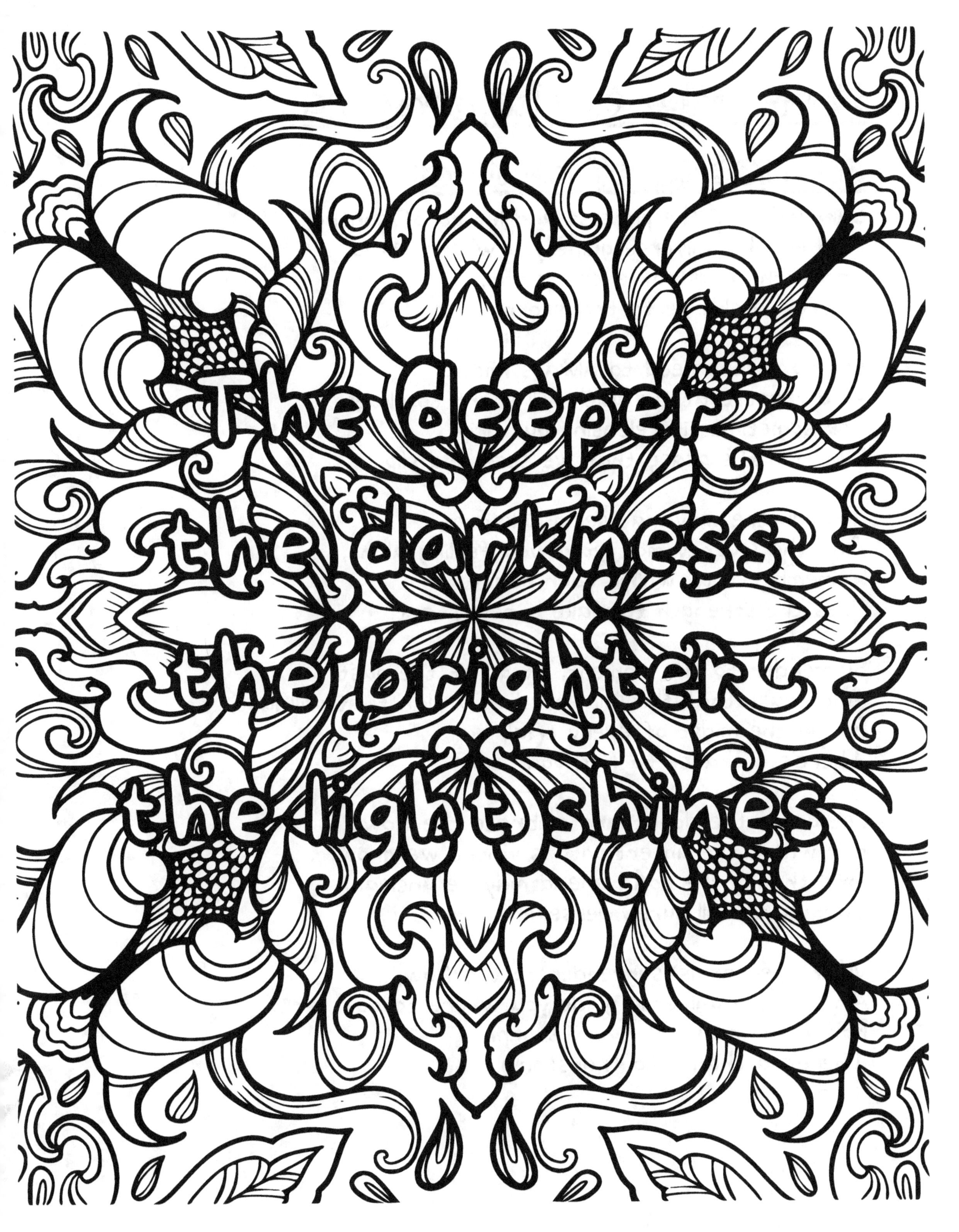

The deeper
the darkness
the brighter
the light shines

Surrender to the process and let go of control

Surrender to the process and let go of control,
And let the universe guide you where to go,
For in the midst of every storm,
There's a chance to transform.

Let go of the need to always know,
And trust that the path will start to show,
For sometimes in releasing our grip,
We find the peace that we seek and slip.

Though the way may seem unknown,
And the journey may leave you feeling alone,
Remember that within your heart,
 Lies the strength to make a new start.

Surrender to the moment, let go of the past,
And trust that the universe has a plan that will last,
For in the midst of every trial,
There's a chance to find your smile.

Let go of the doubt and embrace the flow,
For within the uncertainty is where we grow,
And though the road ahead may be unclear,
Your spirit will surely persevere.

With open arms, surrender to the flow,
And let the universe guide you where to go,
For in the midst of every storm,
There's a chance to transform.

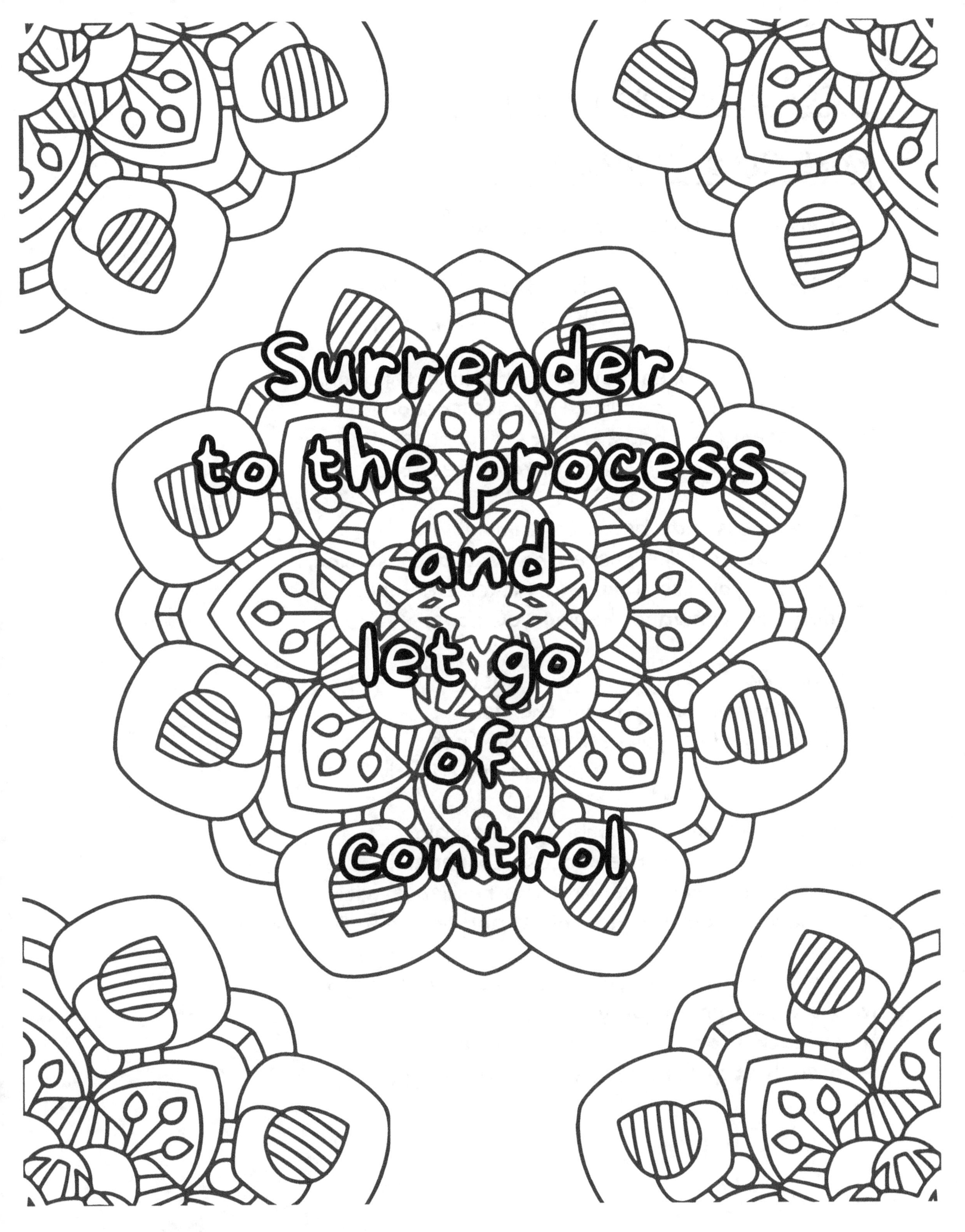

Surrender
to the process
and
let go
of
control

You are not broken
you are breaking through

You may feel shattered, torn apart,
As if your very soul is falling apart,
But listen closely to the beating of your heart,
For it whispers the truth that sets you apart.

You are not broken, you are breaking through,
Like a butterfly emerging from its cocoon,
It may seem like chaos, but it's a process to renew,
To become who you were always meant to.

The darkness may be all-consuming,
And it may feel like there's no way of resuming,
But within you lies a light, a flicker of hope,
Guiding you forward, helping you cope.

You are not a victim of your past,
But a warrior rising from the ash,
With every step, you're breaking free,
From the chains that once held you tightly.

So trust the journey, embrace the pain,
For it's all part of the process to regain,
The strength, the love, and the resilience within,
To emerge from the darkness, and let your light begin.

You are not broken, you are breaking through,
Into a new version of you,
With each scar, you grow stronger,
And each step forward, you'll soar longer.

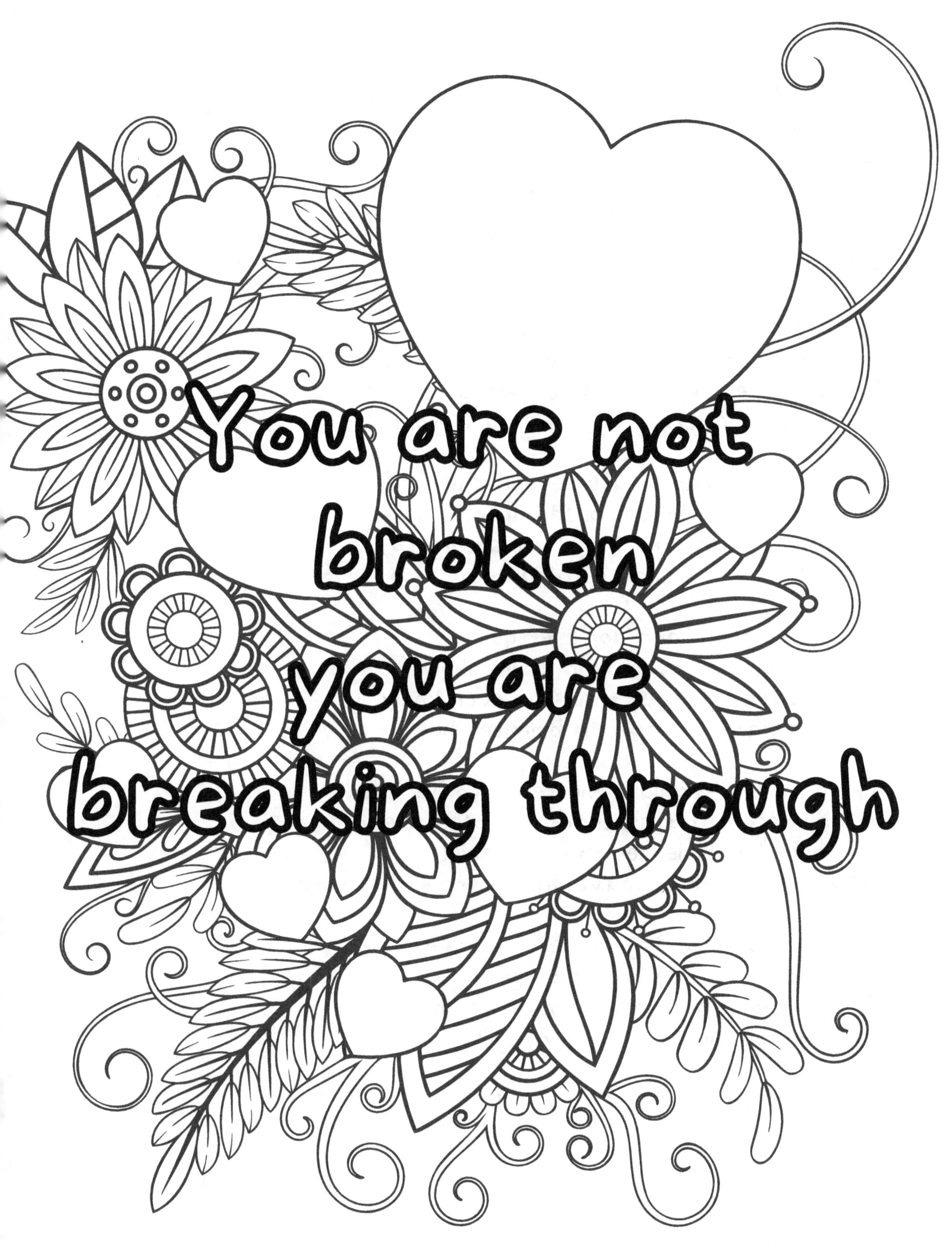
You are not
broken
you are
breaking through

The darkest hour is just before dawn

The night is long, the shadows deep,
And in this darkness, it's hard to sleep,
You wonder if the sun will ever rise,
If hope will ever materialize.

But in this abyss, you're not alone,
For every soul has a darkness they've known,
And just like the stars that shine so bright,
You too, will emerge from this dark night.

The darkest hour is just before dawn,
And soon, the light will break upon,
The horizon, and the world will seem new,
A fresh start, a chance to pursue.

So hold on tight, and don't let go,
For the light will come, and it will show,
That you're stronger than you ever knew,
And the dawn will bring a brighter hue.

The pain, the struggle, the tears you've shed,
Will all become the strength you need ahead,
To face the challenges that will arise,
With the resilience, you've gained from this demise.

The darkest hour is just before dawn,
And soon, you'll see the light upon,
The horizon, and a new day will begin,
Where hope, and love, and joy will win.

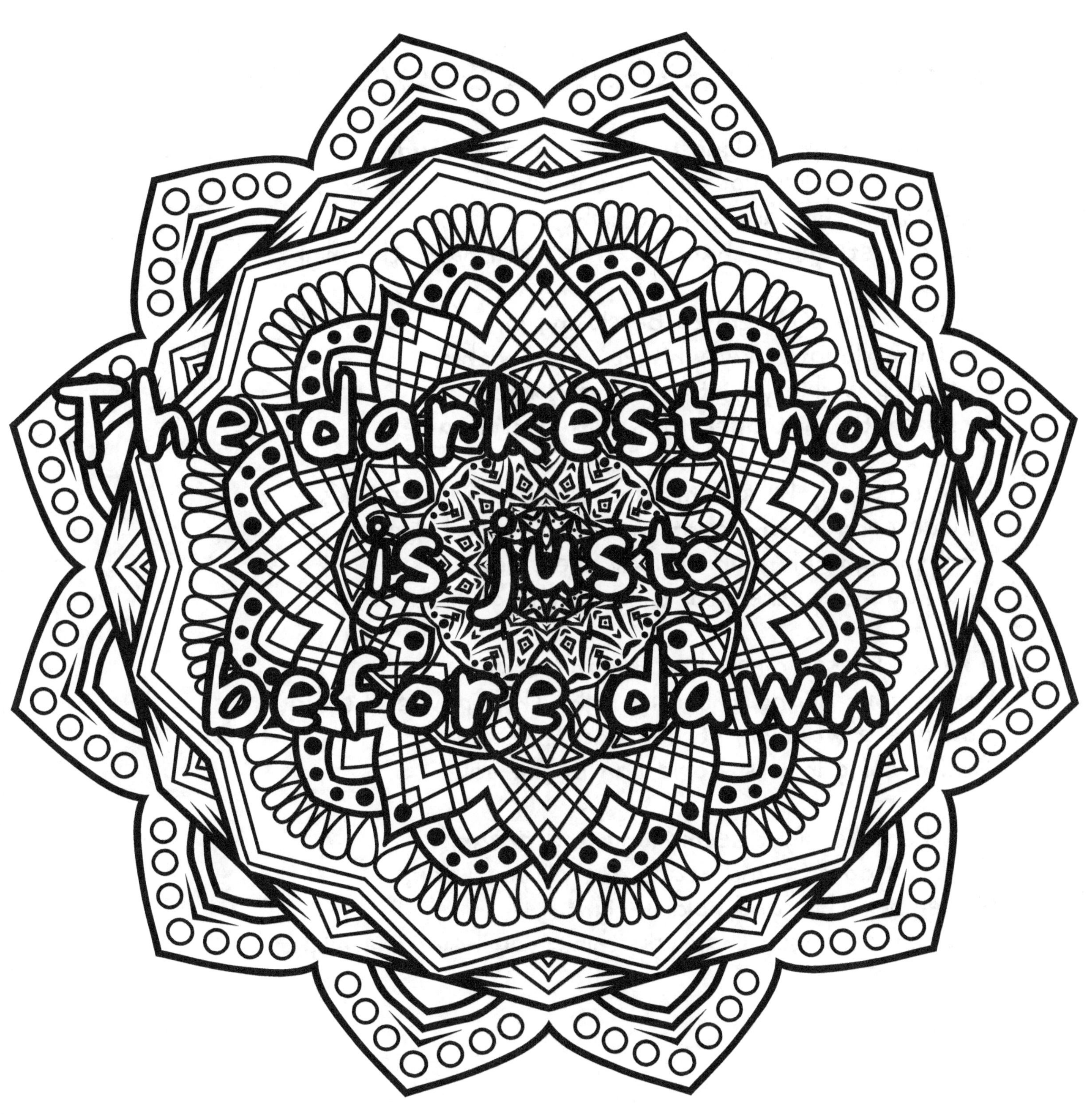
The darkest hour
is just
before dawn

You are stronger than you think

When the night is long and the road is tough,
And you feel like you've had enough,
Remember this, and hold it tight,
You are stronger than you think, you have the might.

The world may seem to be closing in,
And the doubts may whisper from within,
But deep within you, there is a flame,
A strength that burns, it's not just a game.

You've faced the storms and weathered the tides,
You've conquered mountains and crossed divides,
And though this journey may seem hard,
You have the strength, the will, the guard.

The darkness comes, but it can't stay,
For in your heart, there's a light that paves the way,
You are a warrior, strong and true,
And nothing in this world can break you.

So when the night seems long and drear,
And the doubts and fears are all you hear,
Remember this, and hold it tight,
You are stronger than you think, you have the might.

You are stronger than you think

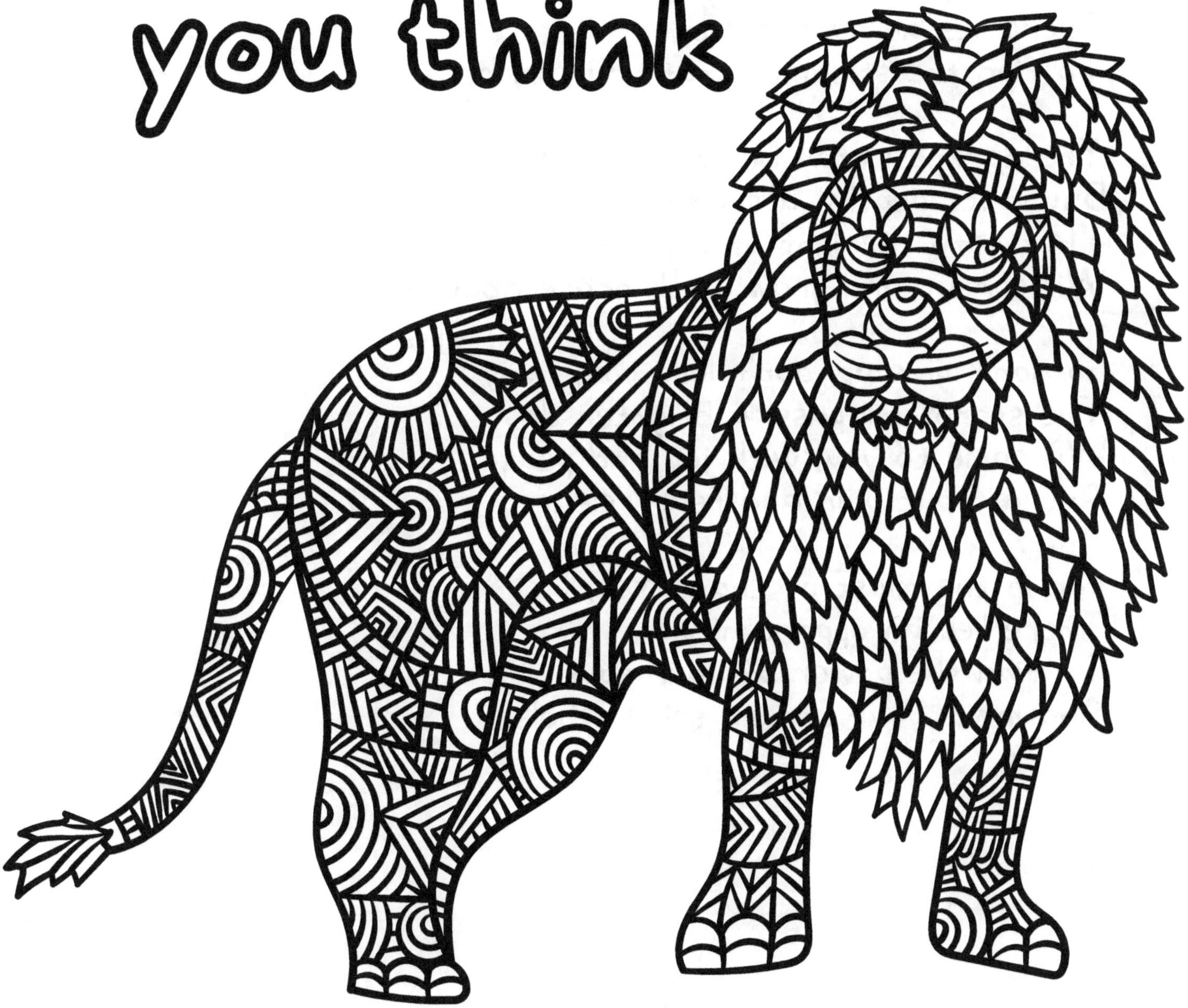

In the midst of chaos there is also opportunity.

Amidst the chaos and the strife,
Amidst the turmoil of your life,
There lies an opportunity,
To find the strength that you can be.

The darkness may be hard to bear,
But in its depths, a seed is there,
That with the light of hope and love,
Will sprout and grow, with grace above.

So don't give up, don't lose your way,
The storm will pass, a brighter day,
Will come to you, with joy and peace,
And all your pain and fear release.

For in the midst of chaos, see,
There lies an opportunity,
To find the power of your soul,
And make your broken spirit whole.

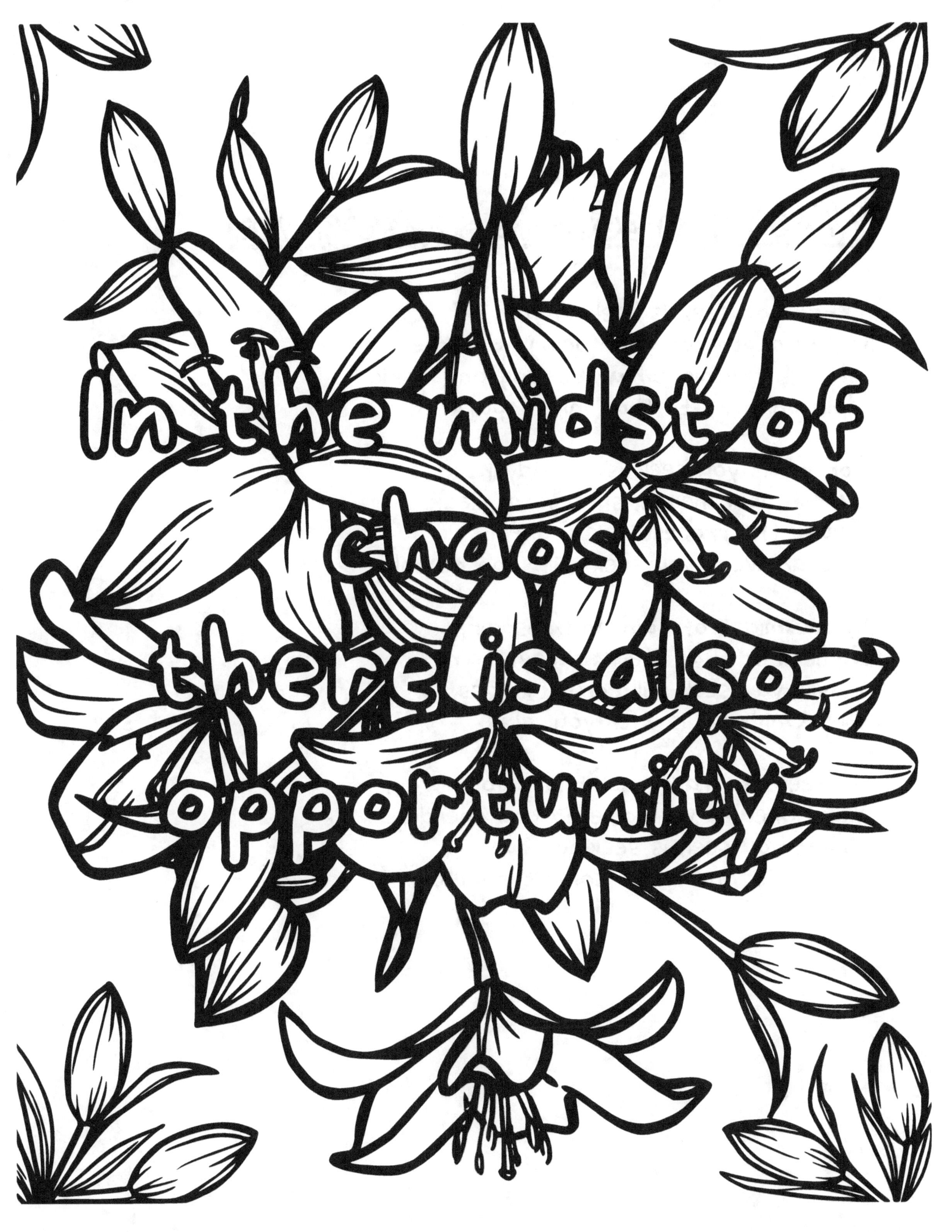

In the midst of
chaos,
there is also
opportunity

What you seek is seeking you

What you seek is seeking you,
In the depths of your being, it's true.
Though the night may be long and dark,
Hold on tight to that inner spark.

For what you seek is already here,
Within your heart, so crystal clear.
Trust the process, let it unfold,
The answers you seek will soon be told.

In the midst of pain and despair,
Remember that life is always fair.
What you seek will come to pass,
The Universe is with you, alas.

So keep the faith, don't lose your way,
Your dreams will come to you one day.
What you seek is seeking you,
Believe it, and it will come through.

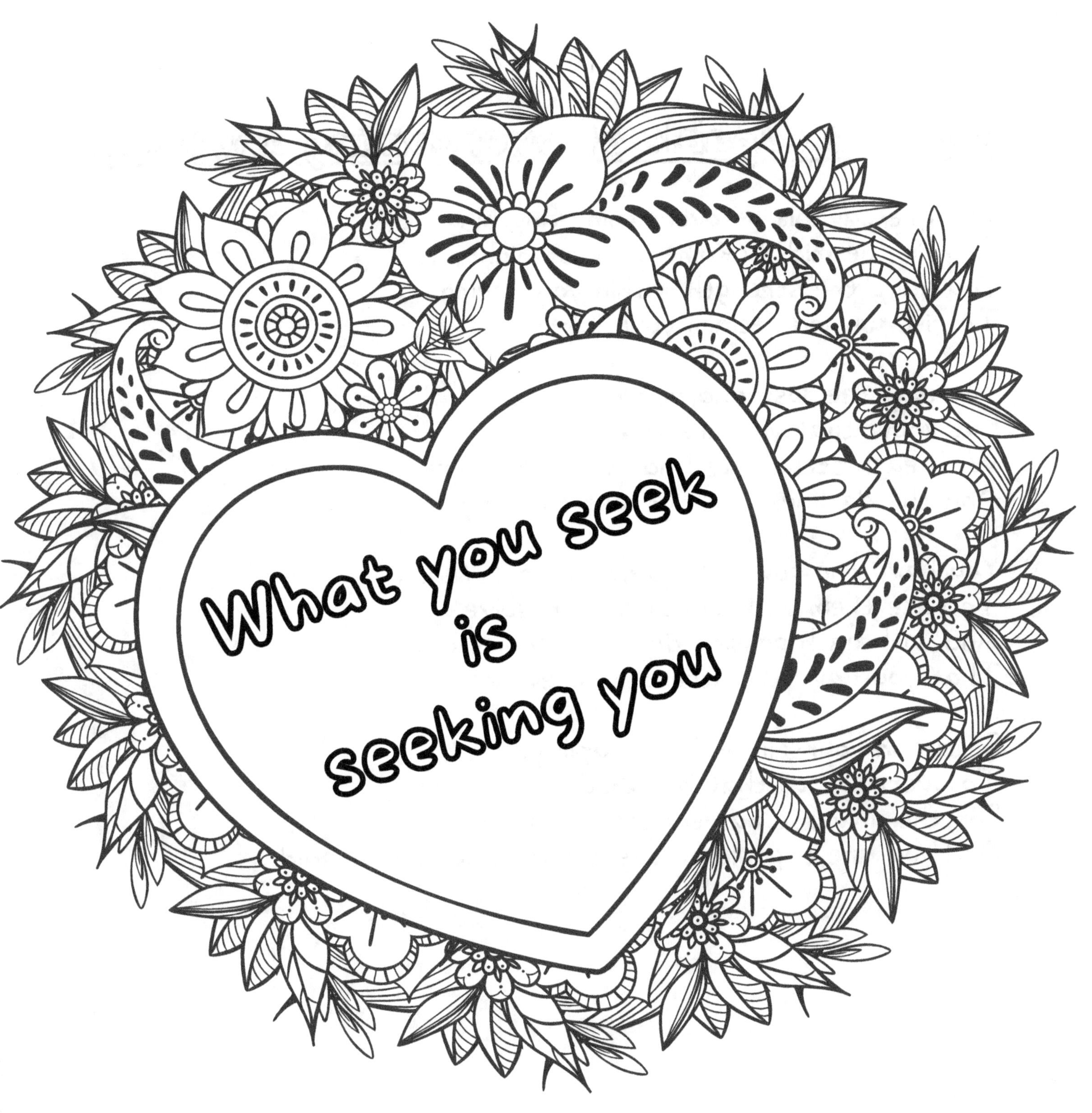
What you seek
is
seeking you

You are capable of overcoming anything

You are capable of overcoming anything,
Even in the midst of the darkest night.
You have the strength within your being,
To rise up and reclaim your light.

You may feel lost and all alone,
But know that you are truly strong.
With each step, you'll find your way home,
And the darkness will not last for long.

You have the power to conquer your fears,
To face them with unwavering resolve.
And with each passing day, it becomes clear,
That you have the strength to evolve.

Believe in yourself and your ability,
To overcome all that lies ahead.
For the universe has endless possibility,
And you are capable of overcoming anything, it said.

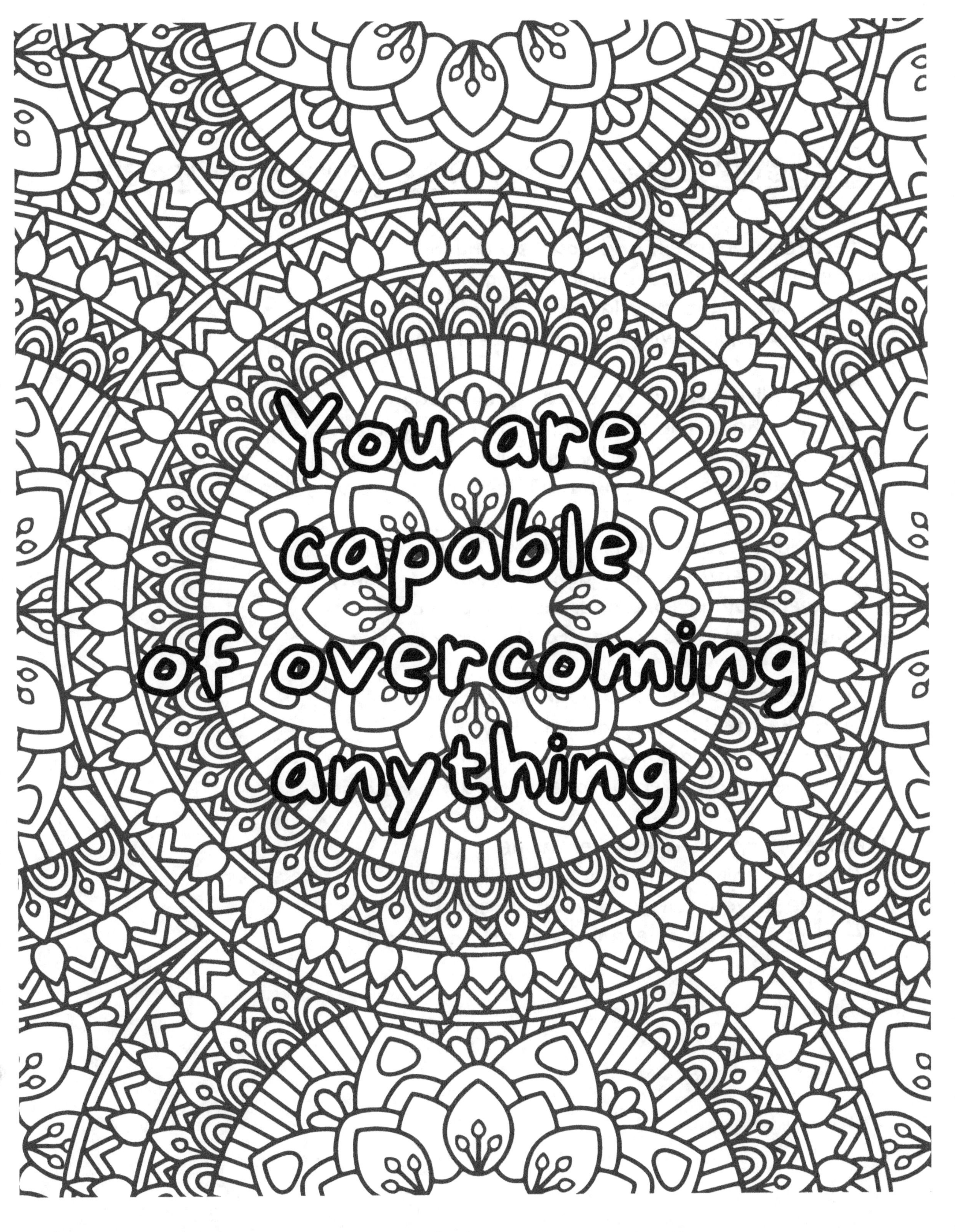
You are
capable
of overcoming
anything

Believe in yourself and your strength

Believe in yourself and your strength,
Even when life seems full of length,
The dark night may last for a while,
But your spirit will never lose its style.

The challenges you face may seem tough,
But you have the courage, and that's enough,
Believe in yourself and your will,
And you'll rise from the darkness, strong and still.

Your inner strength is a guiding light,
That will lead you through the darkest night,
So keep moving forward, don't you stop,
And you'll find your way to the mountain top.

Believe in yourself and your power,
And the light within you will shower,
Through the darkness, you will emerge,
Stronger than ever before, with a new surge.

Remember, you are never alone,
And the universe is your eternal home,
Believe in yourself, and your strength,
And you'll overcome anything, at any length.

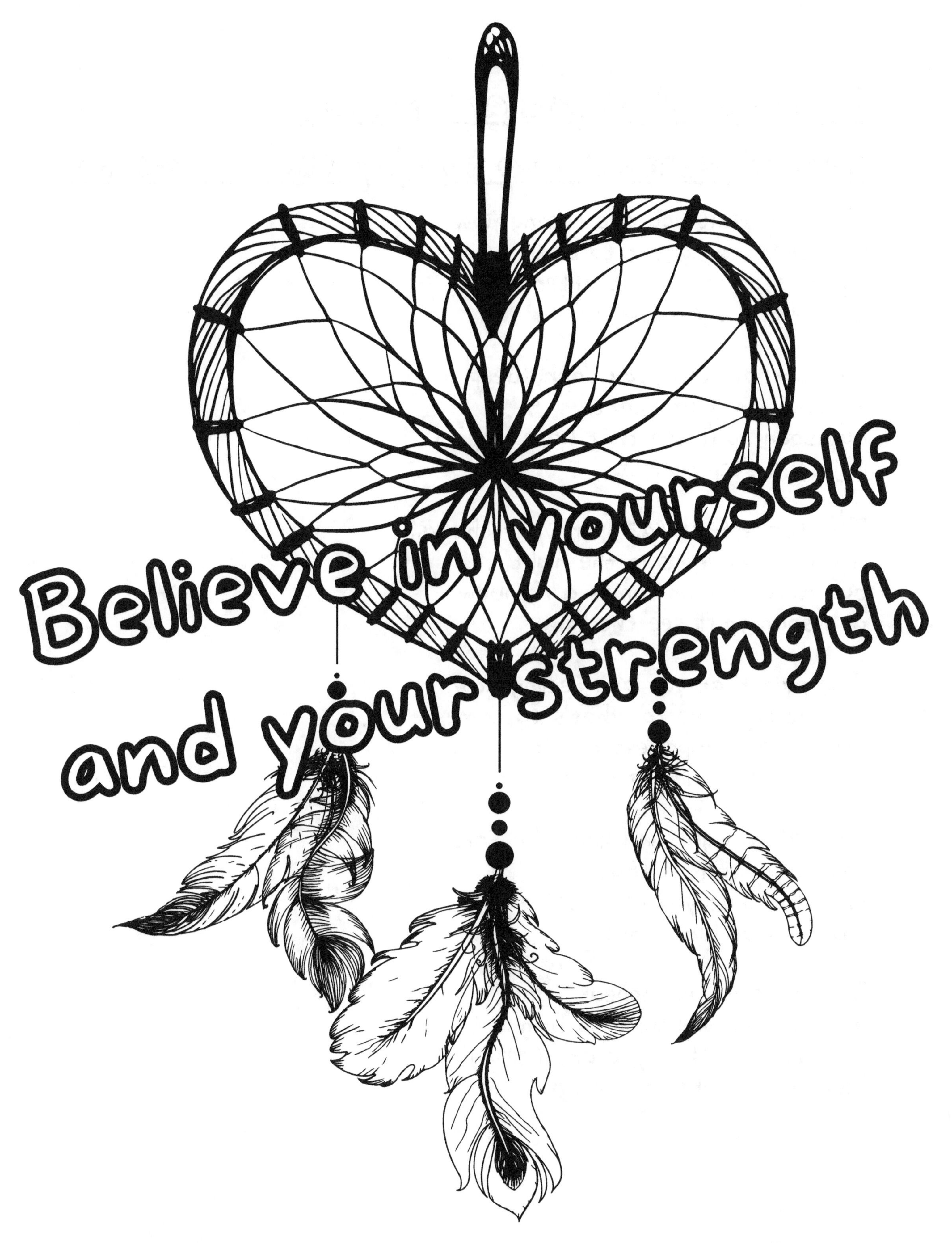

Believe in yourself
and your strength

The pain that you are feeling cannot compare to the joy that is coming

The pain that you are feeling now,
may seem too great to bear,
but keep in mind that after dark,
the light is everywhere.

The sorrow that you carry deep,
is heavy on your heart,
but soon you'll see that happiness,
is just a step apart.

The tears that fall upon your cheeks,
are like raindrops in the night,
but after storm comes a rainbow,
and soon you'll see the light.

The pain that you are feeling now,
cannot compare to what's to come,
for joy and happiness await,
when your healing is done.

So hold on tight and keep the faith,
believe in what is true,
the pain that you are feeling now,
will soon be but a hue.

The rainbow will appear again,
and the sun will shine so bright,
for the pain that you are feeling now,
cannot compare to the light.

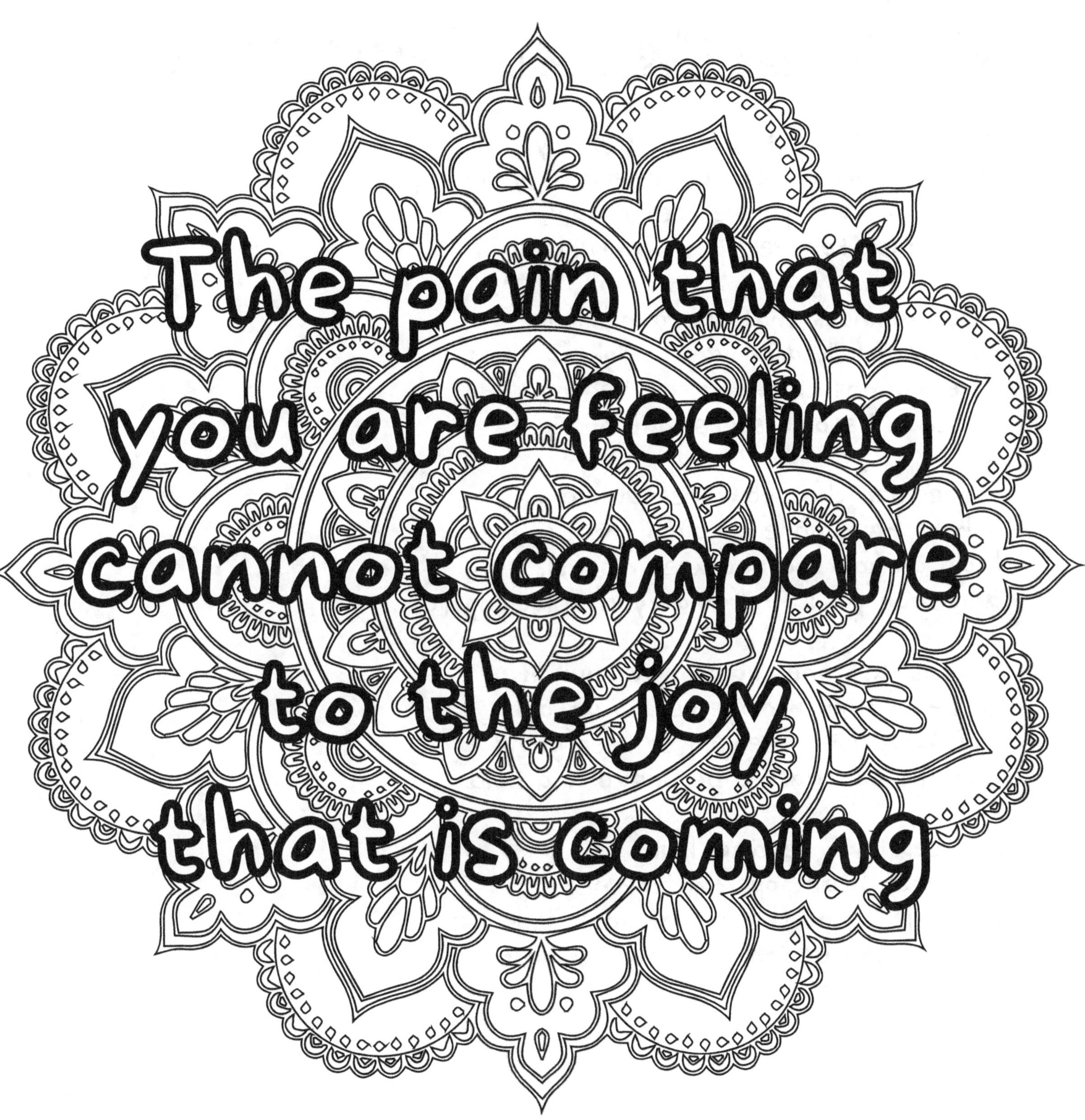

The pain that
you are feeling
cannot compare
to the joy
that is coming

This is not the end of your story.

This is not the end of your story,
though it may feel like the end of your world.
The pain that you're feeling now,
won't last forever, it will unfurl.

The darkness that surrounds you,
will eventually give way to light.
The wounds that you are healing,
will soon become scars, out of sight.

Remember that you are not alone,
others have gone through this before.
Hold on to hope and keep moving,
and soon you'll find what you're looking for.

This is just one chapter of your life,
there's so much more yet to unfold.
You have the strength to keep going,
and the courage to be brave and bold.

So keep your head up high,
and your heart open to the new.
For this is not the end of your story,
it's just the beginning of something true.

This is
not the end
of your story

Keep going even when it's hard

In the depths of night when all seems lost,
And the path ahead is shrouded in frost,
When the weight of the world feels hard to bear,
And it seems like nobody else is there.

Remember this, my dear and true,
That every step you take is one towards the new,
 And though the road is steep and rough,
You must keep going, even when it's tough.

For there is always light beyond the dark,
And every storm will pass, leave its mark,
The struggles we face make us strong,
And teach us lessons that will last long.

So keep your head up, eyes fixed ahead,
Take each day as it comes, no need to dread,
Believe in yourself and all that you can be,
And keep going, even when it's hard to see.

For the journey ahead may be winding and long,
But with each step you take, you grow ever strong,
And the trials that once seemed so immense,
Will become mere memories in the future tense.

So keep going, dear one, through the dark of the night,
For the dawn will come and bring new light,
And the struggles you face will make you whole,
Keep going, even when it's hard to hold.

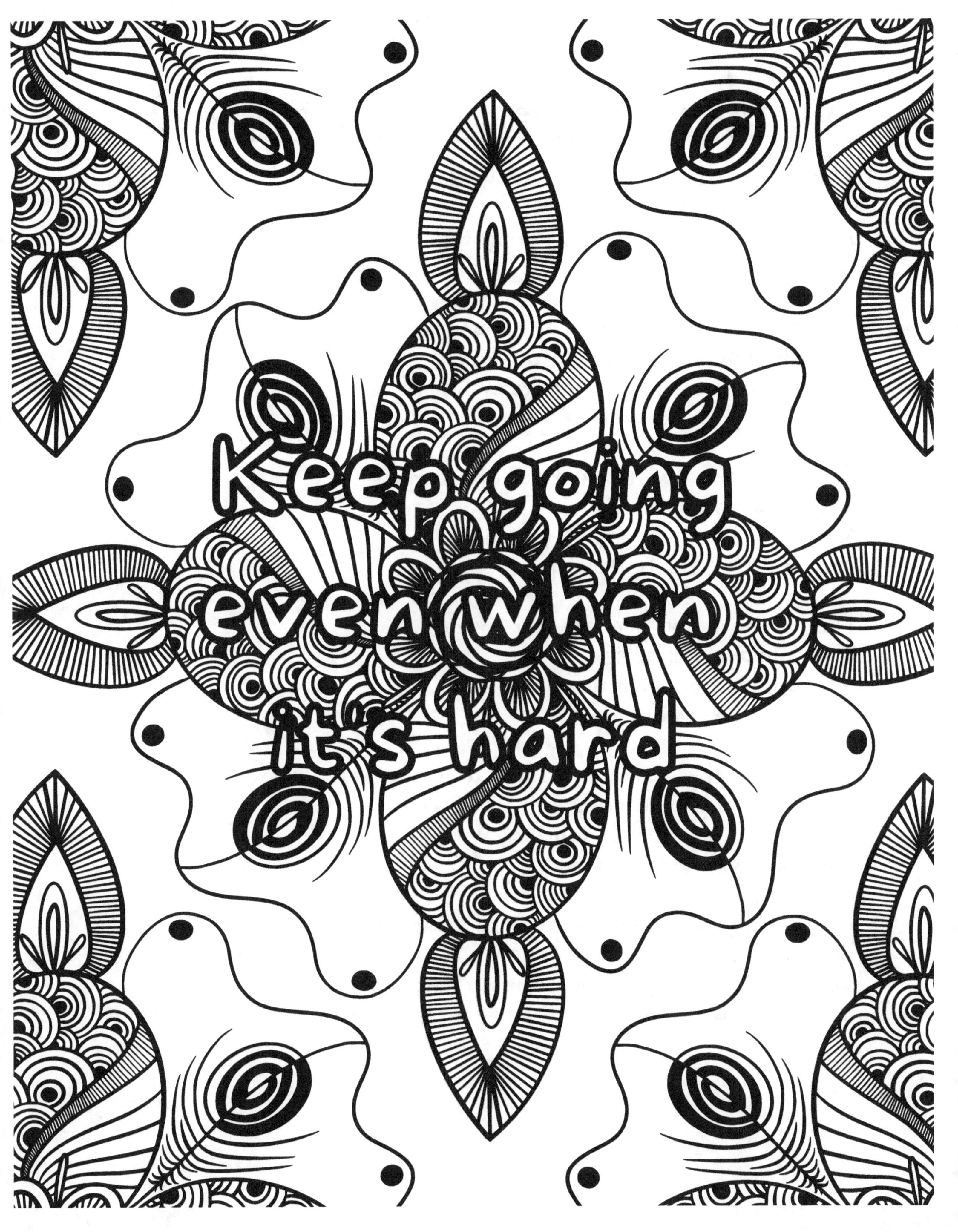

Keep going
even when
it's hard

Stay strong even when it's tough

When darkness falls and shadows loom
And hope seems out of sight
When life becomes a heavy weight
And everything's a fight

Stay strong, my friend, stay strong and true
Though troubles weigh you down
For in your heart there beats a flame
That's brighter than a crown

The road may twist and turn and bend
And trials may abound
But know that you are not alone
And help can still be found

The strength you need is deep inside
And courage will arise
Hold on, hold on with all your might
And lift your weary eyes

For though the storm may rage and roar
And skies may turn to grey
The sun will rise again someday
And light will find its way

Stay strong, my friend, stay strong and true
And do not be afraid
For though the night may seem so long
A brighter dawn is made.

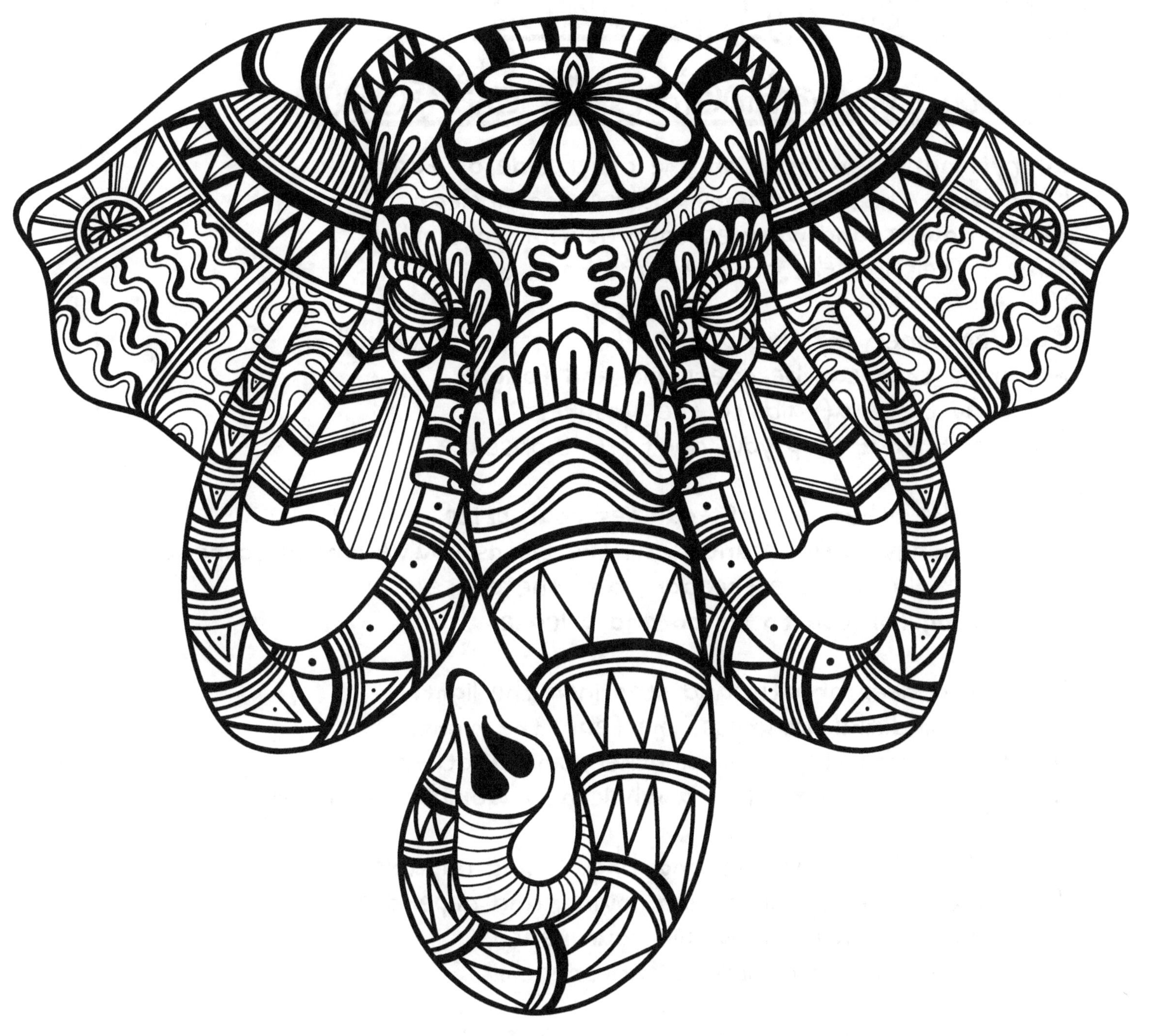

Stay strong even when it's tough

Everything you want is on the other side of fear

Everything you want is on the other side of fear,
Even when the night seems endless and unclear,
When doubts and worries take hold of your mind,
And it feels like the answers are hard to find.

But remember, my friend, that fear is just a thought,
A hurdle that can be overcome and fought,
It's okay to be afraid, to feel unsure,
But don't let it stop you, don't let it obscure.

For on the other side of fear lies your prize,
All the things you've wanted, all the things you've longed to realize,
The love, the joy, the freedom, and the peace,
All waiting for you to let go and release.

So take a deep breath, and step into the light,
Leave behind the darkness, the fear, the night,
Take one small step, then another, and another,
Soon you'll find yourself in a whole new world of wonder.

Remember that you're strong, brave, and capable,
And that the universe is kind, loving, and dependable,
Everything you want is within your reach,
All you have to do is believe and breach.

So go on, my friend, take that leap of faith,
Embrace the unknown, the new, the great,
For everything you want is on the other side of fear,
And it's waiting for you to show up, and draw near.

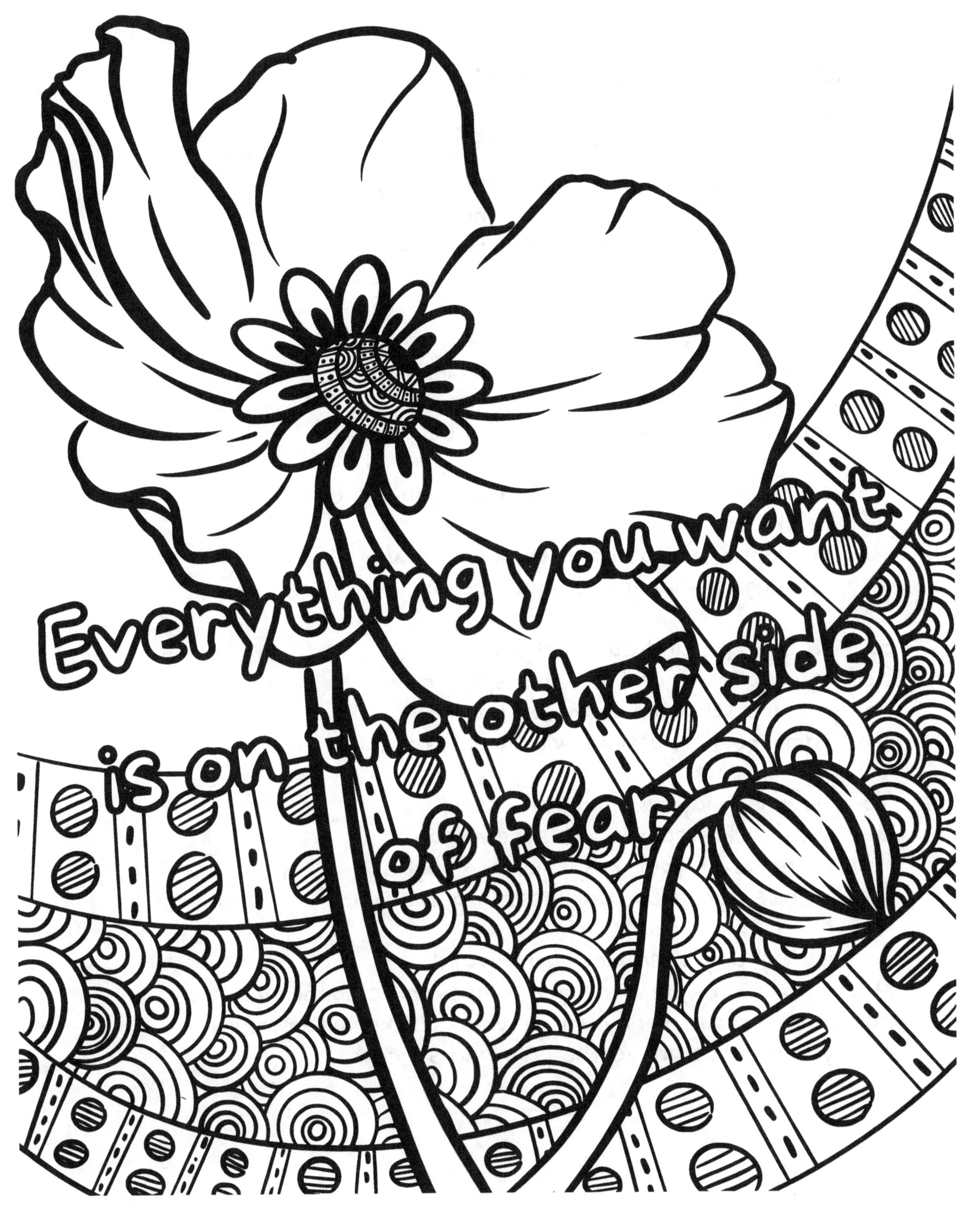

Everything you want is on the other side of fear

<u>Your struggle today</u>
<u>will be your strength tomorrow</u>

When the weight of the world feels heavy on your chest
And life's challenges put you to the test,
When the tears won't stop and the pain won't cease
And your heart feels like it's lost in the seas.

Remember that your struggle today
Will be the strength that guides your way.
For every hurdle that you overcome
Is a step towards the person you'll become.

The scars you bear and the battles you fight
Will be the fuel that ignites your light.
And though it may be hard to see it now,
Your struggles will become your crown.

So hold on tight and don't let go,
Believe in yourself and let your spirit glow.
For you are stronger than you know,
And tomorrow's blessings will surely show.

Your journey may be tough and steep,
But with each step, you will surely reap
The rewards of your resilience and might,
As you rise above the darkness into the light.

So keep fighting, keep moving forward,
And know that your strength will never be cornered.
For your struggle today will be your strength tomorrow,
And you will rise above the pain and sorrow.

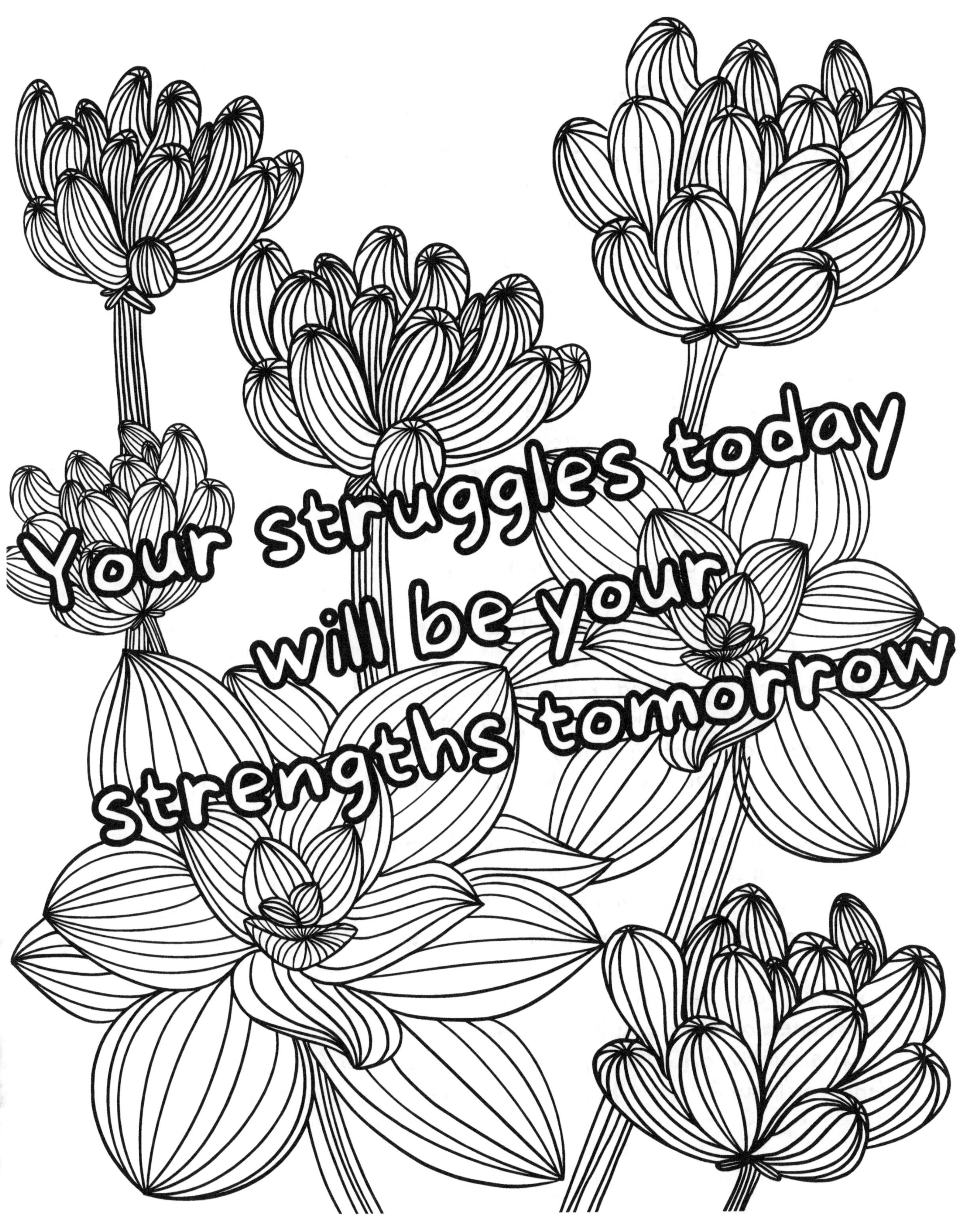

Your struggles today
will be your
strengths tomorrow

You have survived 100% of your worst day so far

You have faced the darkest nights,
And felt the weight of crushing frights.
You've been knocked down and felt the pain,
But through it all, you've still remained.

You've walked through fire, and braved the storm,
You've weathered all that life has formed.
You've seen the worst that can befall,
And yet, you're standing still, tall.

So know that you have what it takes,
To conquer all that comes your way.
You've survived each test and trial,
And grown stronger with each denial.

Take heart, my friend, for you have proven,
That in the end, you'll keep on moving.
You'll keep on fighting, and keep on striving,
Until you've reached the other side, surviving.

For you have faced your worst with grace,
And in your heart, you'll find the space,
To overcome the darkest days,
And find the strength to light your way.

So when you feel you can't go on,
Remember all that you have done.
You've survived 100% of your worst days so far,
And you'll survive the rest, with courage in your heart.

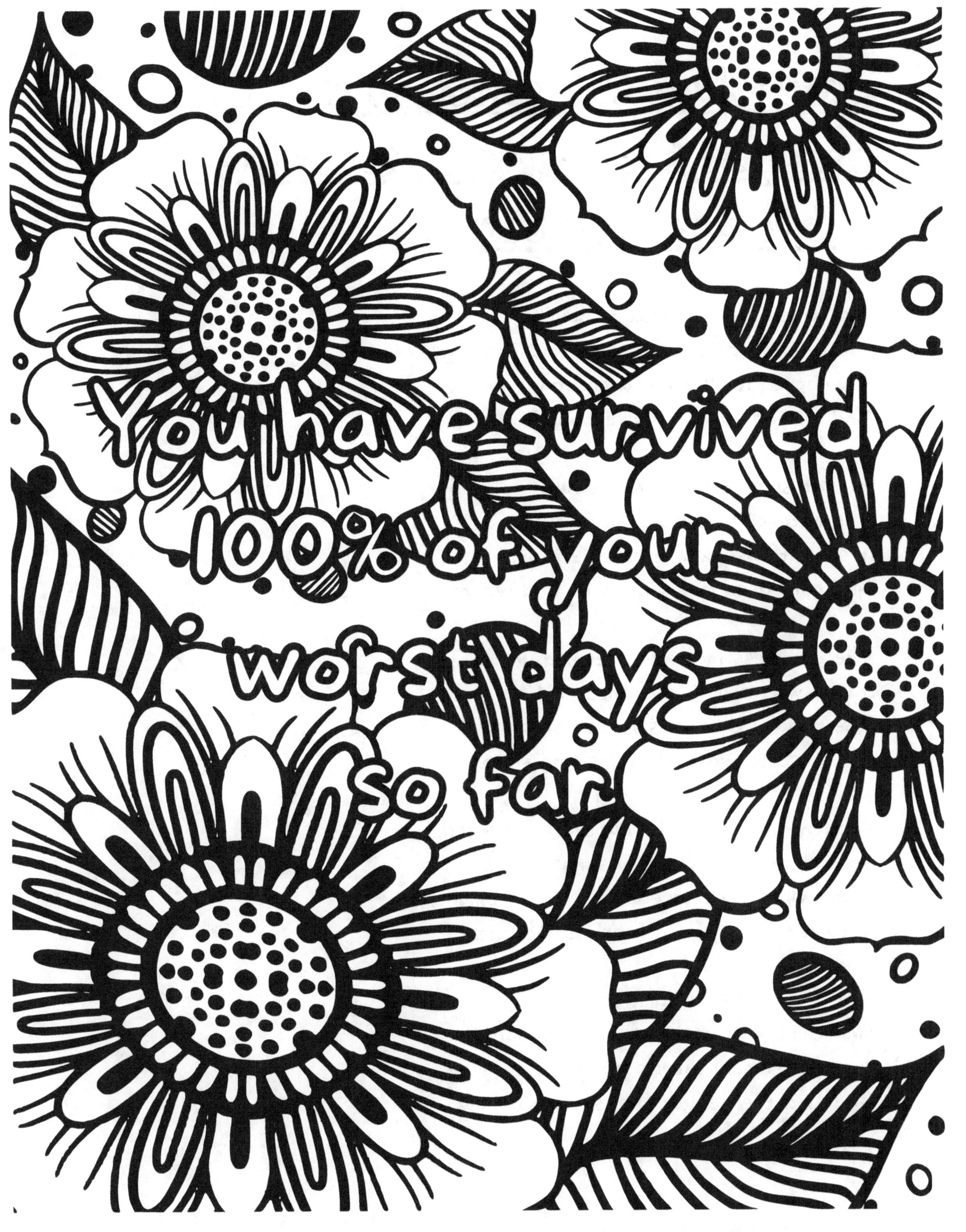
You have survived
100% of your
worst days
so far

<u>Just when the caterpillar thought the world was ending, it became a butterfly</u>

Just when the caterpillar thought,
The world was ending, bleak and fraught,
It wrapped itself up in a cocoon,
And waited for its darkest moon.

In that space of pain and doubt,
The caterpillar turned inside out,
It shed its old skin, its former form,
And embraced a change, wild and warm.

The darkness may have seemed unkind,
But it was a gift, a chance to find,
The beauty that was hidden deep,
A chance to wake from its long sleep.

And then one day, the butterfly emerged,
A thing of beauty, newly surged,
With wings that spread and colors bright,
It took to the sky, in fearless flight.

So if you are in a dark cocoon,
And think the world will end you soon,
Just remember, there's a chance to grow,
And find the beauty that's yet to show.

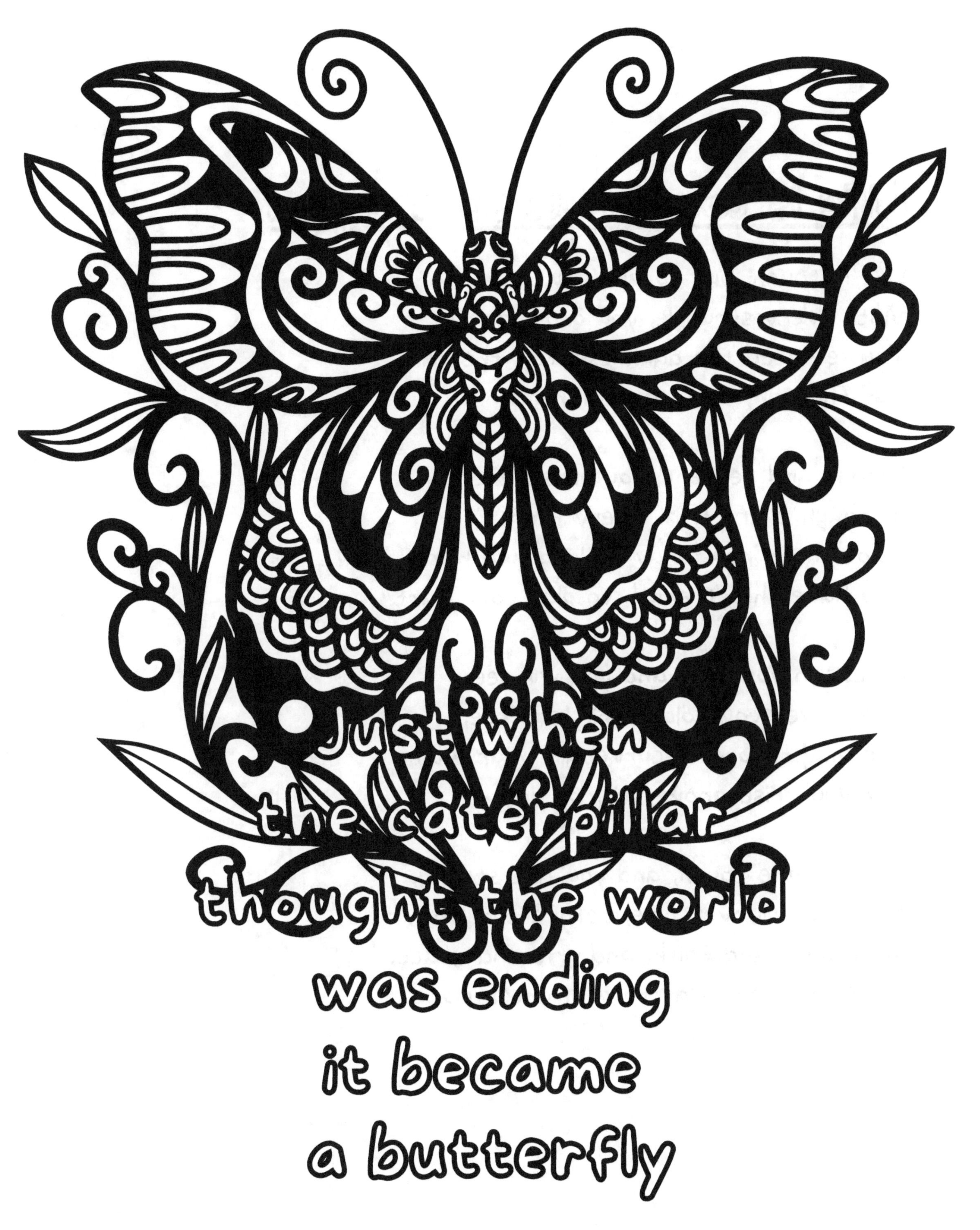

Just when
the caterpillar
thought the world
was ending
it became
a butterfly

Life is tough but so are you

Life is tough, but so are you,
With every struggle, you grow anew,
You've faced the darkness, felt the pain,
But through it all, you still remain.

Strong and resilient, you persevere,
Through every trial, every fear,
Though the road may be long and hard,
You have the strength to play your part.

Believe in yourself, and you will see,
The power you hold within, so free,
Life may throw its curveballs your way,
But you'll rise above, day by day.

For you are tough, and you are strong,
And you will overcome, before too long
With hope and faith, and grit and grace,
You'll find your way to a brighter place.

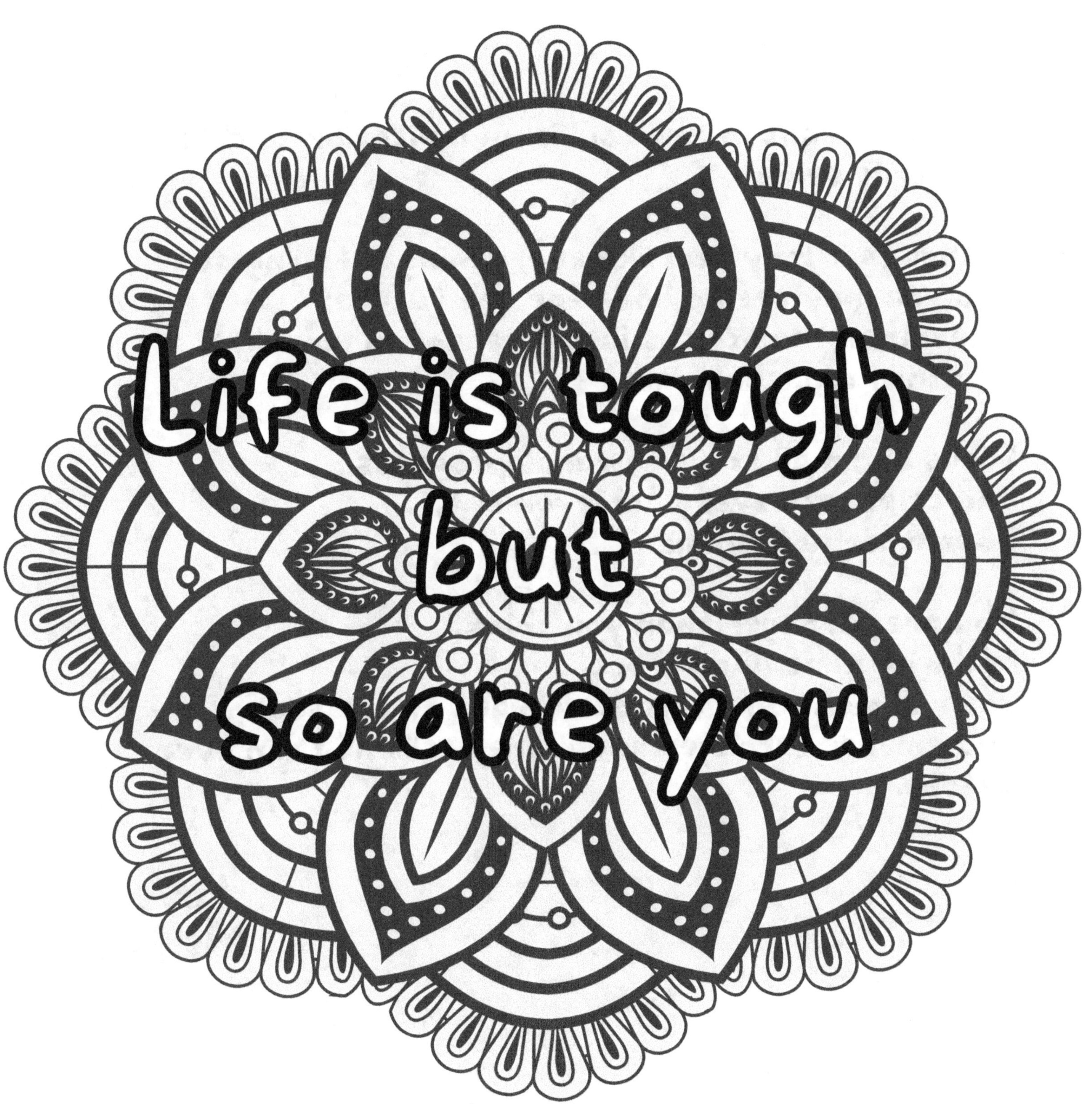

Life is tough
but
so are you

The dark night of the soul is an invitation to discover
your true self.

Although it may feel like everything is falling apart,
and you may see no hope for the future;
remember that this is just a season in your life,
and this, too, shall pass.

Focus on small steps towards progress,
and celebrate every achievement,
no matter how small.

You are stronger than you think,
and with time and effort,
you will overcome this dark night of the soul,
and emerge stronger and more resilient than ever
before.

Love,
Ms.Egg